Migraine Reset

Seth H. Evans, MD

Copyright © 2019 Seth H. Evans, MD

All rights reserved.

ISBN: 9781794050822

DEDICATION

To Audrey Evans, as you are just over one year into your life's journey. You bring me the greatest of joy every day, and I can't wait to see what the future holds.

CONTENTS

	Acknowledgments	i
1	A New Paradigm	11
2	First Things First	23
3	Status Quo	35
4	State of the Art	45
5	Target the Source	61
6	Know the Past to Know the Present	73
7	Migraine RESET	83
8	Frequently Asked Questions	95
9	Ending Thoughts	109
10	Resources	113

ACKNOWLEDGMENTS

I would like to thank all the teachers I had through my many years of school and training, but especially my mentors at Virginia Commonwealth University.

I thank my parents, Bobby and Pam Evans, for their unwavering support for me and my dreams, and the solid foundation they provided for my life.

And finally, I thank my partner and best friend, Renee Evans, for her faith in me, her dedication to us, and her constant drive to be the best version of herself.

Chapter 1:

A New Paradigm

Seth H. Evans, M.D.

1 A NEW PARADIGM

The day when it all began started just like any other workday. This particular day was sometime back in early 2016. I was seeing the typical mix of ear, nose and throat patients in my office, no different than usual.

Somewhere in the middle of the morning, I stepped into an exam room to meet a new patient to my practice. This was a very nice lady who was in her mid-30s. The first thing I noticed was that she looked downright miserable. She complained mainly of a severe headache which had lasted for over one month without any relief. The pain was nearly unbearable and would not ease, even for a few minutes. She had a many-year history of migraine headaches, which had become more and more severe over time. Finally, this most recent headache had lasted for over one month.

During her month of misery, she had already been to the emergency room several times and had been given various pain medications and other anti-migraine medications without any relief. Several CT scans and MRI scans were used to see inside her head, but all of them showed normal findings except some mild areas of inflammation in her sinuses.

She was now coming to see me (in desperation) because she was told that her headache might be caused by either a sinus infection or something wrong with her sinuses. After I was able to evaluate her and review her CT scan, I realized that there was nothing wrong with her sinuses and that her headache was caused by a severe and intractable case of migraine.

Normally, as an ENT specialist, that would be the end of my involvement for this unfortunate lady. I could confidently say that her sinuses were not the issue and send her back to her neurologist for further evaluation.

However, this day was different.

I'd recently started learning about a new treatment for migraine headaches: a treatment for which my specific knowledge and skills as an ENT doctor were especially relevant.

Now, you may stop and ask yourself, "Why is an ear, nose and throat doctor interested in treating migraine headaches? I thought that neurologists treat migraines." That is true, but we ENT doctors see patients with migraine ALL THE TIME. The reason we see so many migraineurs (that's a fancy term for someone who gets migraine headaches) is that symptoms of migraine can frequently mimic ear, nose, and throat conditions. These include sinus problems, dizziness, ringing in the ears, and other conditions that are in the realm of the ENT specialty. As a specialist in this field, I end up seeing a lot of patients with migraines even though they come to me thinking they have another problem.

So, to make a long story short, I decided to offer my patient the new treatment that I recently learned about. You'll hear much more about this treatment in the second half of the book. To offer a bit of a teaser: the treatment is a very simple procedure, which is performed by me in the office. It usually takes 30 seconds or less, start to finish. It involves placing medication into the inside of the nose. It is not painful (but does feel a bit weird). It has zero risk of any serious complications. Most patients have no side effects, but some people will have brief mild side effects after the treatment for 1-2 hours. For someone who suffers from severe migraines, this treatment can potentially provide life-changing relief. It is a true game-changer for many.

Back to the story... I finished evaluating my patient and explained my assessment and recommendations for her. I decided to offer her the new treatment, and she agreed to try it. This treatment, again, is very simple for someone with my training to perform. After I did it, I left the room for a few minutes and then came back to see if there had been any effect.

I asked her, "How are you feeling?" She said, "I don't feel anything." When she said this, I felt a little bit let down. I assumed that she meant that nothing happened from the treatment and her headache was still raging on like it had for the past month. I think she realized that and hastily added, "No, no, I don't feel the headache anymore. It's gone." I just stared at her for a moment, in a bit of shock. I think she was a little stunned herself that this terrible headache that had been present for over a month was now suddenly gone.

Obviously from my side of things, I was delighted and encouraged by this initial result and dedicated myself to learning more and more about this new treatment and how I could best use it to help people who suffer from migraines and many other painful conditions.

So, I'm guessing by this point, you are thinking "What *IS* this new treatment??? Tell me what it is!" Don't worry, we'll get to that! As you read onward into this book, I'm going to be telling you a lot more about this treatment, which I have further developed and refined. I've fine-tuned what I think is the best, quickest, and easiest way to perform it. I call my specific method the <u>RESET Treatment</u>.

The RESET can be used to relieve an active migraine headache and to prevent future migraines. In addition, it can be used to treat a number of other types of facial pain syndromes or headaches, as well as types of pain that occur in other parts of the body. These include chronic neck and back pain, as well as sciatica.

Why is it called RESET? Well, the letters stand for Relieve & Eliminate Symptoms Endoscopic Treatment. The other reason I call it RESET is because it acts like hitting the reset button on pain, specifically headaches. If you ever had a problem with your computer or another electronic device, usually hitting the reset button will fix the problem. This analogy works well for migraine headaches and other conditions that are helped by this treatment.

What does this treatment involve?

In a nutshell, the RESET treatment consists of using local anesthesia (i.e. numbing medication) to block a nerve located inside your nose. I use a thin endoscope to see inside of your nose. This endoscope looks a bit like a thin metal straw, and it contains a fiberoptic cable that I can use to see places in the back of your nose that are not visible any other way.

In the very back of the nasal cavity, above where your nose joins into your throat, there is a small nerve bundle called the sphenopalatine ganglion. This nerve bundle lies on one of the major nerve branches that provides sensation to the face and the rest of the head. As a result, the nerve signals that transmit the unpleasant pain of migraine headaches travel through this area. Using the small endoscope to see, I'm able to precisely squirt numbing medicine over this nerve bundle and thus, block the nerve's function.

This nerve block does several things. First, we can potentially relieve a migraine headache that's currently happening. But not only that, we also can prevent headaches in the future with the RESET treatment! How long this beneficial effect will last is variable among different patients, but the benefit can last weeks to months in some people. The RESET treatment is not painful and it has no serious risks.

Interestingly, the treatment of blocking the sphenopalatine ganglion has been around for over 100 years. It was first developed and performed in 1909. There are various different methods that have been developed to perform the treatment. The particular way that I perform it using a thin nasal endoscope for visualization is unique to my own practice (to my knowledge). Although some other ENT doctors may have also started offering this treatment, I haven't seen another ENT publicizing this online (as of the date of publication of this book).

How did I learn about this treatment?

I originally discovered the treatment through an advertisement that was sent to me for a medical device called the SphenoCath. This device is designed to blindly inject the numbing medicine into the nose to block the sphenopalatine ganglion. It made out of soft material and is bent at a certain angle to help facilitate getting the numbing medication into the correct spot. I realized very quickly that as an ear, nose and throat specialist, I didn't need this device and I could perform the treatment much more accurately using my endoscope to see inside of the nose. I also realized what a huge population of suffering migraine patients could be helped by this type of treatment!

Nasal endoscopy is a procedure that I routinely perform multiple times every day in my office and I am very comfortable and experienced with looking and working inside of people's noses. As I started learning more about what I now call the RESET treatment, I also re-educated myself about migraine and what a terrible disease it is. After what I've learned, I count myself very fortunate to have never experienced the pain and misery that migraines cause for so many people.

I also started learning about the typically inadequate treatment and lack of relief that most patients with migraine receive. I will talk a lot more later on in this book about why I believe this is happening and how patients can get better treatment for their migraines.

Why should you read this book? What will you gain?

The biggest benefit for someone with migraine who's reading this book is the potential to relieve your pain and your headaches. The RESET treatment provides unbelievably good outcomes in many patients. People who've had the terrible problem of migraines for many years can actually get true lasting relief. Try to imagine walking around pain-free if you've been having migraines several times a week (or every day!) for years on end. Imagine not having to worry about a migraine rearing its ugly head at the worst time, maybe right in the middle of a friend's visit or when your child has a performance that you wanted to go see.

So many people have to deal with headaches happening all the time and they're always having to make excuses and go lie down to deal with their migraine. Even if the migraines aren't completely eliminated by the RESET, it is quite possible that you can have less frequent headaches or less severe headaches with this treatment.

What are the downsides of not reading this book?

The biggest downside is not learning about a treatment that can relieve your pain. You may end up with continued long-term pain from having migraine headaches. In addition, as anyone with migraine knows, nausea is typically associated with the headache. Sometimes the nausea and vomiting can be worse than the headache! It's hard to work and even harder to think when you're having a migraine. And even if you're home, you'll likely suffer from decreased quality time with your family and friends.

The worst thing about migraines is their close association with mental illness like depression. There is sadly a high risk of suicide in patients who suffer from frequent migraines. It's somewhat understandable that if someone's in such severe pain over and over again, life can be pretty bleak. But if this treatment can help even one person step back from that dark place, I'll happily keep performing it as long as I am able to practice medicine.

What will the reader learn?

This book is divided into two parts. In the first half of the book, I will review the current knowledge of migraine headaches, what they are and how they happen. We'll then discuss what most people are doing now to try and treat their migraine headaches (spoiler alert: it's not pretty). Finally, we will learn about what is considered "state-of-the-art" treatment for migraines today. This includes many different medications, but also a large number of lifestyle changes including diet, exercise and other non-medical treatments.

The second half of this book will be an in-depth discussion of the RESET treatment: what it is, its history from the early days over 100 years ago up to the present. Finally, we'll learn what I have done to optimize and improve this treatment and how it can help you to get relief from your migraine headaches.

Contact Information:

If you live in the Austin area, you can reach my office to schedule an appointment at texanent.com or 512-550-0321. If you live elsewhere or wish to see another doctor, I have a short video that teaches other ENT doctors how I perform the RESET treatment at texanent.com/video-for-doctors.

Seth H. Evans, M.D.

Chapter 2:

First Things First

Seth H. Evans, M.D.

2 FIRST THINGS FIRST

What is the definition of a migraine headache?

I can tell you it is not what most people think. Most folks (and this includes many doctors!) have in their minds that all migraines are the same. Here's the typical story: First, when someone starts to develop a migraine, they'll start by seeing flashing lights. Then, the headache will start pounding and will keep going all day, while the poor person lies down in their dark bedroom, praying for it to pass. During the headache, there's nausea and vomiting and just generally feeling awful. Now, many migraines are like this, but this is not how they always happen by any stretch. There is a wide spectrum of migraine symptoms that can be very different from this "classic picture."

For migraine headaches specifically, there are diagnostic criteria which were published by the International Headache Society (IHS). If any recurrent headache meets these specified criteria, then by definition, it is considered a migraine.

The first rule is that the headache must last <u>longer than four but less than 72 hours</u>. Second, patients should have at least two out of these four criteria:
1. The headache is on one side only.
2. The headache has a pulsating quality, meaning that it feels like the head is throbbing or pulsing back and forth.
3. The headache is moderate to severe in intensity.
4. The headache becomes worse with routine physical activity such as walking up a flight of stairs or carrying groceries.

The next part of the definition is the headache must be associated with at least one of these two things: nausea or photophobia. Photophobia is sensitivity to bright lights. Finally, other causes of the headache need to be ruled out. If a patient meets those specific criteria, by definition, they have a migraine headache. You may notice that there was nothing about visual changes or lights flashing in any of that definition. We'll discuss the reason for that shortly.

Are migraines only headaches?

The answer is no. In the past few years, the concept of migraine has shifted away from just a bad headache to become a full body neurologic disorder. Specifically, it is a disorder of abnormal sensation. Obviously, the most important one of those abnormal sensations is pain in the head, but there can also be other abnormal sensations. Common examples of these include dizziness, ringing in the ears, abdominal pain, and many other problems.

Another difficult thing for migraineurs is that other illnesses or problems tend to feel worse for them. This is because of the abnormal sensory inputs seen in migraine patients. What would be a mild case of dizziness for someone else can be an incapacitating dizziness for someone with migraine disorder. Things just feel worse when you are prone to migraines (even if you are not currently in the middle of a headache).

What are the two main subtypes of migraine?

The two subtypes are <u>migraine with aura</u> and <u>migraine without aura</u>. In the "classic picture" of a migraine headache, the aura is the lights flashing or visual changes that happen before the onset of the headache. Although migraine with aura is considered the classic picture of this disease, only about 20% of all migraineurs have an aura preceding their headaches. In contrast, the vast majority of about 80% do not have an aura preceding their headache. And not all auras are visual in nature. The most common aura is changes to vision including flashing lights or blurring, but there can be many other sensory or other neurological disturbances. It can include things like a phantom smell or taste, severe dizziness, and even other neurologic symptoms like seizures or mini strokes.

What are common misdiagnoses that are really migraines in disguise?

There are many types of headaches and other symptoms that are actually caused by migraine but are misdiagnosed routinely as other conditions. A very common one that I see all the time as an ear, nose and throat specialist is sinus headache. Sinus pressure and discomfort is generally not caused by a sinus infection unless there is also nasal congestion, thick discolored drainage from the nose, and loss of smell. Isolated pressure and pain in the sinuses without these additional nasal symptoms is much more likely to be a result of migraine.

Many patients are convinced, however, that their sinuses are the problem. It is easy for people to get confused because the pharmaceutical industry profits off of selling special "sinus headache" medications such as Tylenol Cold and Sinus. The problem is these medications all help migraine as well, so just because your headache gets better after taking a "cold and sinus" pill does not prove that anything was wrong with your actual sinuses.

Another common misdiagnosis is tension headache. This type of headache is just what it sounds like. These headaches are purported to be caused by tension within the scalp and muscles of the forehead. They commonly occur after a stressful day, a poor night of sleep, or when you get dehydrated. It is suspected, though, that these tension headaches are really a more mild form of migraine rather than truly caused by muscle tension. The idea is that the muscle tension is caused by the (migraine) headache, rather than the headache being caused by the muscle tension.

A non-headache symptom that is frequently caused by migraine is dizziness or vertigo. This is another symptom that I see all the time as an ear, nose and throat specialist because people assume there's something wrong with their ears if they're having dizziness. Migraine is probably the most common cause of dizziness in most people and can seem very much like an inner ear problem at times. There are also many other symptoms throughout the body that can actually be attributed to migraines, including ringing in the ears and abdominal pain (this is especially common in children).

What is the cause of migraine?

The exact mechanism for why migraines happen and how they happen is not known. Although lots of neuroscience research has been done, unfortunately, we still don't truly understand how our brains work or why they do the things they do. So, the answer to the question of what is the true cause of migraines is "we don't know."

There are, however, helpful mental models for people to understand how migraines happen and what people can do to prevent them or treat them.

One very useful model is the Triggers and Threshold model. This idea is described in great detail in the book Heal Your Headache by Dr. David Buchholz. The fundamental idea with this model is that everyone actually has the mechanism in their brain to get a migraine if they reach a certain threshold. Most people's threshold is far too high for them ever to have a migraine headache. But for patients who get migraines, their threshold is much lower.

This is where the idea of triggers comes in. As people accumulate more and more triggers, they are pushed higher and closer to their individual thresholds for migraine. Triggers can be lots of different things: allergies, dehydration, hormone changes, lack of sleep, many different foods and drinks. All of these things can build on each other. If the amount of triggers get high enough to reach over a certain person's threshold, they will develop a migraine headache.

What happens physiologically with migraine?

Migraine headaches start with a build up of one or more triggers. Perhaps you got a poor night of sleep last night, endured a stressful meeting with your boss at work in the morning, and then drowned your sorrows with a glass (or three) of red wine with dinner. You may have set off a migraine with this combination of triggers. Each one alone might have not caused any problem, but the combination adds up to push you over your threshold.

In an unknown way, these triggers activate a part of the brain deep inside the center of your head called the hypothalamus. Our modern understanding is that this area of the brain starts the dominoes falling that result in a full-blown migraine headache. The hypothalamus releases signals that result in something called cortical spreading depression (CSD). Despite the term "depression," CSD is counterintuitively a wave of electrical excitatory energy, which spreads over the outer surface of the brain (called the cerebral cortex).

The next step in the cascade is activation of a large nerve that supplies sensation to the face and the head called the trigeminal nerve. The trigeminal nerve is a major nerve within the head. It has multiple important functions including transmitting sensory information from the head and the face back to the brain, but also sending out autonomic nerve signals from the brain to the surrounding tissues.

As the migraine headache starts, it is the outward-bound autonomic nerve fibers that send the message "Start the Headache!" to the tissues in the rest of your head. The end result of this signaling is that the blood vessels in the lining around the brain and elsewhere in your head and face start to dilate and become inflamed.

When this happens, pain signals are generated in the inflamed blood vessels. These signals then make a quick U-turn and zip back up the trigeminal nerve to the brain. The pain sensation is then processed by your brain and felt in your conscious experience as a migraine headache.

A bit of foreshadowing: we now know about the trigeminal nerve, what it is, and its central role in migraine headaches. This nerve is the main two-way signaling pathway for migraines- carrying instructions from the brain outward, and then transmitting pain signals inward. As a result, the trigeminal nerve is an excellent target for stopping migraine headaches in their tracks and preventing them in the future.

Who gets migraines?

Migraine headaches are extremely common. About 20% of all women (and post-pubescent girls) in the United States suffer from them. Around 5% of men and 5% of prepubescent children also have migraine headaches. There are approximately 38 million total people in the United States who get migraines. This is 12% of the total population. 25% of all households contain someone who gets migraines. Migraine headaches are most common between the ages of 25 and 55 years old, but can happen at almost any age. Finally, 90% of patients who get migraines also have a family member who gets migraines.

What are the economic costs of migraines?

About 90% of patients with migraines are unable to work or function effectively while they're having a headache. Unfortunately, our American culture is not very sensitive or forgiving for migraineurs. Many people feel intense pressure to struggle through work, but are less effective in their job performance. As a result, the performance of the business they work for suffers. The average migraineur has one to two headaches per month, but a lot of patients have many more than that.

There are four million people in the United States who suffer from chronic daily migraine. This condition is defined as having more than 15 headache days per month. But it can truly be every day for some unfortunate people.

About every 10 seconds someone in the United States goes to the emergency room for a headache. There are a total of 1.2 million emergency room visits every year for migraines. All of this adds up to a massive amount of lost economic production and an equally huge amount of money spent on healthcare. If migraines could be treated better, especially by preventing them in the first place, maybe some of this money could be saved for better uses.

What are the costs to each individual patient?

Obviously, migraines cause horrible pain. No one wants to be feeling that type of pain. In addition, there's the nausea, which is commonly associated with the headaches. I'm fortunate that I've never suffered from a migraine headache, but in my experience, there is no feeling in the world worse than nausea and vomiting. Sometimes I might think the nausea can be even worse than the pain of the headache.

Then there are the associated conditions of migraine including depression, anxiety, and other mental problems. On top of all this is the unstated expectation that migraineurs just have to keep working or care for their family anyway. All of this can make people feel really awful.

So, we've begun our journey through the current knowledge of migraine disorder in this first chapter. You're now up to date on the most current understanding of what migraines are, the mechanism of how the headaches start and transmit through the head, and the terrible burden they place on individuals and our society as a whole.

We'll now move on to learn about what can be done for this massive problem. The next chapter will discuss what most people end up doing, and as you'll soon find out, it's not ideal.

# Chapter 3:

Status Quo

Seth H. Evans, M.D.

3 STATUS QUO

One sobering statistic to start this chapter: over 50% of all migraineurs never go to a doctor for treatment of their headaches! For such a severe problem that affects so many millions of Americans, it is quite surprising that so few end up seeking medical care. I think there are a few reasons for this statistic. One major issue is that there are an endless supply of over-the-counter migraine medications, such as Excedrin migraine or others of the same ilk. Most of these medications work ok, especially for infrequent or less severe migraines, but when overused, they can lead into a vicious cycle of rebound headaches.

Are most people reactive or proactive?

This is a simple matter of human psychology. Most people are reactive in nature most of the time (myself included). What is the difference between reactive and proactive? Well, reactive people generally wait for something to happen to them and then they try and deal with it. Proactive people, on the other hand, try and think ahead to what might happen and take steps to deal with it or prevent it before it happens. As a matter of typical psychology, most people (if they're already feeling okay) are going to just wait and react to the moment rather than trying to plan ahead for all eventualities.

For this reason, the majority of people who get migraines usually just attempt to treat their headaches once they occur. But they're not necessarily doing anything to try to prevent the headaches in the first place. There are some quite significant long-term downsides to this style of managing headaches, as you'll find out.

What are the most common treatments for migraines?

The number one treatment for most people is over-the-counter medication. These types of medicine include things like Excedrin migraine or Advil migraine. There's usually the word migraine within the brand name, to make it obvious for the consumer. All of these medications can be effective, but they're usually not sufficient for people with more severe or more frequent migraines. And all of them can lead to more frequent headaches in the long run. For someone with infrequent headaches, once or twice a month (or fewer), these medications can be quite helpful.

The majority of patients with migraines unfortunately try to treat their condition by themselves. I think there is a general consensus among many migraineurs that there is no good treatment and that their condition is not curable. They become resigned to their destiny, and just try to endure the headaches as best they can.

Add to that fact, many doctors are not exactly thrilled to see a patient for migraines. Doctors know as well as anyone that the most common medical treatments used for migraines don't work very well. Most of us doctors got into medicine to help people, and it is hard to feel like you can't help someone. As you'll learn in the next chapter, there are actually a lot of options to prevent and manage migraines, but these options usually take a lot of time (for the patient and the doctor) and education of the patient to be effective. In today's healthcare climate of packed schedules and 7 minutes per patient, a lot of docs are just not able to do anything except write a quick prescription and run on to the next patient. Because of this, the care for migraine patients (and many others) suffers.

Ok, I'll get off my soapbox...

Many migraineurs do go to their doctors, though, and there are a number of prescription medications that can also treat headaches. These include medicines called triptans, which block a specific serotonin receptor in the brain. By blocking this receptor, the resulting inflammatory pathway can be temporarily blocked, leading to lessened pain and constriction of blood vessels in the head.

In addition, stronger medicines like opioids can be used to treat the pain of migraines. Opioids include medicines like morphine, dilaudid, demerol, or hydrocodone. These medications are quite strong but are purely used to block pain, and are not actually stopping the migraine pathway. Obviously, opioids also carry significant risks of addiction as well as overdose.

Then there is another medication called Fioricet, which contains Tylenol, butalbital (a sedative) and caffeine, which can block migraine headaches. Fioricet can work very well, but again, like all these other options it can lead to worse problems if used too frequently.

All of these most commonly used medications are reactive (or abortive) treatments for migraine. People take them when they feel the headache is starting (or once it has already started). These medications don't prevent headaches from happening.

What is a rebound headache?

A rebound headache is exactly the same as a regular migraine headache. The difference is that the trigger for the rebound headache is the withdrawal off of a medication used to treat the previous headache. Why does this happen? The reason is all of the medications that are used to block migraines cause constriction of blood vessels. If you remember back to the previous chapter, when a migraine happens, there's dilation of blood vessels throughout the head and facial area. Because of this fact, medications that constrict these blood vessels can block or eliminate the headache.

The problem is once the medication wears off, the blood vessels rebound and dilate open again and then the headache comes roaring back with a vengeance. This usually does not happen if abortive medications are only used once or twice a month.

Rebound headache is possible if a patient uses these types of medications more than twice a month and the risk increases more and more as these medications are used more frequently. Many patients can use these types of medicines more often without a problem, but the more they are used, the more risky it becomes.

In fact, the most common reason that migraine headaches increase in frequency is the overuse of abortive medications like triptans, fioricet, non-steroidals (like aspirin or ibuprofen), or opioids. As a result of this overuse, there is an increase in rebound headaches and it creates a vicious cycle. The patient is getting more and more rebound headaches, so they're using more and more abortive medications and things just get worse and worse.

Do most people seek help from a doctor for migraines?

No, as we already said earlier, most people don't. The majority of all migraineurs are usually trying to treat themselves with over-the-counter medications. Some will end up going to doctors, but a lot of times these are not migraine specialists. They're either primary care doctors or acute care providers who work in urgent care centers or the emergency room. I'm not saying that these are bad doctors, but they're not necessarily the experts in long-term migraine treatment. Any doctor can educate themselves, but most overworked docs are unable to spend much time doing this.

Some patients, however, will end up seeing a neurologist, who's typically considered the specialist for migraines. But even many neurologists don't have a particular interest in migraines and don't take a lot of time to create the ideal treatment pathway for migraine patients. So fewer still will end up finally seeing a neurologist who has true interest and expertise in headache management. Now, these patients will probably end up getting good treatment (or at least good recommendations). But unfortunately, it is few and far between that anyone is able to see these types of headache specialists.

Who are the traditional specialists for migraine?

Traditionally, most would consider the expert in migraines to be a neurologist, especially a sub-specialist who has completed extra training in headache treatment. However, as I said before, many neurologists have different interests and are less interested in treating migraine and other types of headache.

In addition, in recent years, pain medicine doctors have also taken an important role in treating migraines and other types of headache and facial pain. These specialists are experts at treating and relieving pain throughout the body, including pain in the head from migraines.

However, many patients with migraine will still end up seeing other specialists, especially for some of their alternative symptoms. As an ENT doctor, I frequently see patients with "sinus headache", which are really migraines, as well as dizziness and ringing in the ears. All of these symptoms can result from migraines, not actual sinus or ear problems.

Gastroenterologists can see patients with abdominal pain and nausea that are related to migraine. Ophthalmologists see patients with visual auras that they may be having due to migraine. Orthopedic surgeons and neurosurgeons may end up seeing patients with back or neck pain that are related to their migraines.

Migraine is a great mimic of other conditions, and it can be quite difficult to distinguish it from a variety of other problems throughout the body.

Do the majority of migraine patients get optimal treatment?

In my humble opinion, no. Unfortunately, migraine is a difficult problem to treat. At least, it's always been seen that way by most doctors and patients. Again, with basic human psychology, it's easy for patients to give up and think there's never any good options for them. On the other hand, it's also easy for doctors to give up on these patients because despite their best efforts and their best knowledge, too many migraine patients just don't get better.

Are you depressed yet? I hope not, because this book is about to start moving in a happier direction. We'll head on now to talk more about the state of the art migraine management of the 21st century. As you'll learn, there are actually a lot of options out there for patients with severe migraines.

Chapter 4:

State of the Art

Seth H. Evans, M.D.

4 STATE OF THE ART

I like to think about migraine treatment sort of like one of those giant all-you-can-eat buffets at a big Las Vegas casino hotel. Stay with me here for a minute. If you've never been to one, it is certainly quite the experience. These buffets are massive, and there are usually well over 100 food options for you to attempt to shovel into your stomach. You will definitely not leave hungry if you ever decide to try one of these places out!

Why do I think of a Vegas buffet when I think about the options for migraine treatment? Well, because there are an equally huge number of options available for treating migraines. And just like every person has different preferences for the food on a buffet, every individual migraine patient will respond differently and prefer certain treatment options over others. There are a wide variety of different medications used to treat migraines and many options for non-medical therapy as well. The combination of treatments may be widely divergent for one patient versus another to get the same improvement.

As we start our overview of the current understanding of "best" treatment for migraines, let's start with a little review.

What is threshold?

We'll return to our mental model for understanding migraines. This model is laid out in much more detail in the book Heal Your Headache by Dr. David Buchholz. Again, his theory is that everyone has a certain threshold or setpoint over which they will develop a migraine headache. If enough triggers pile up until they reach their threshold, then the patient will develop a migraine. As more and more triggers pile on over the threshold, the migraine gets worse and worse. In most people, however, their threshold is too high for them to ever actually have a migraine. Migraineurs have a lower threshold, and thus, have the ability to suffer from the headaches.

What are triggers?

Triggers of migraine can be almost anything and they can be widely variable among different individuals. In some patients, a certain trigger may cause a migraine. In other patients, that exact same thing may actually help a migraine. Probably the biggest trigger is changes in hormone levels, especially those that occur during the menstrual cycle in women. This is the main reason that migraines are 4 times more common in women than in men or children. It is a frequent occurrence for women to have migraines around the time of their menstrual period, but it can also be triggered by other hormone fluctuations during their menstrual cycle, such as ovulation.

During pregnancy, there are also a huge amount of hormone changes. A lot of times, women can actually have improvements in their migraines during pregnancy, especially during the 2nd and 3rd trimesters. In other women, the headaches will become worse during this time.

Diet also plays an extremely important role with many different foods or drinks that can trigger or cause migraines. Caffeinated drinks are probably the #1 offender in this category. We'll discuss other common food and drink triggers later in this chapter.

Lack of sleep is a huge trigger for migraines. It's really important that patients with migraines get good quality sleep every night or they're very likely to suffer the next day. It's recommended that migraineurs get at least 7-8 hours of sleep every night (easier said than done, I know!).

Stress is another big one. If you have a very stressful day, it can easily trigger a migraine. Weather or changes in barometric pressure can also trigger migraines for many people. Finally, allergies or different seasonal changes can trigger migraines. There are many more of these triggers and to list them all would be beyond the scope of this book.

What are the two main categories of migraine medications?

The two categories are abortive and preventive. Abortive medications are those which you take when you get a migraine. The point of the medication is to make the headache go away. Preventative medicines on the other hand are medications that you should take regularly (usually everyday) to prevent the headaches from happening or at least lower the number of headaches that occur.

What are typical abortive medications?

The most common abortive medication that's prescribed by doctors is a class of medications called triptans. These medications are called this because "triptan" is in the name of all the drugs. The original medication in this class is sumatriptan (brand name is Imitrex). Other common ones that are prescribed are zolmitriptan (Zomig), elitriptan (Relpax), rizatriptan (Maxalt), and various others.

Triptans are medications that attach to and stimulate a specific serotonin receptor in the brain. By doing this, they have the effect of blocking inflammation and also constricting blood vessels in the head and neck. As a result, the migraine headache is relieved. Triptans are powerful drugs and can work very well, but like all abortive medications, they can cause rebound headache if they are used too often. If they are used more than twice a month, there is a risk of rebound headache.

Another common abortive medication would be a class called nonsteroidal anti-inflammatory drugs or NSAIDs. These medications are typically over-the-counter and include medicines like ibuprofen or naproxen. They can be helpful especially for milder migraines, but may not be strong enough for more severe or frequent migraines.

Fioricet, which is a medicine containing Tylenol, butalbital, and caffeine can be used for severe headaches, but also has a very strong rebound headache risk. Opioids like morphine, dilaudid, or hydrocodone can also be used for very severe headache pain and a lot of times they are used in the emergency room for patients with migraine.

Finally, there's a class of medicine called ergotamines. These medications are typically used in hospitalized migraine patients when all else fails. Again, all these abortive medications carry a risk of rebound headache and actually making the headaches worse with time. They should not be the primary treatment for migraine headaches (though all too frequently they are).

What are preventive medications?

These are medicines that are taken on a regular schedule to help prevent migraines from happening. All of these preventive medicines were originally developed for another use. Thus, they are considered off-label in use for migraine prevention. "Off-label" use of a medication is not anything bad, it is very common in all medical specialties. Common examples of off-label use would be using aspirin (a pain reliever) to lower risk of heart attack or using benadryl (an allergy medicine) to help treat insomnia. The point of all the preventive medications is that they should raise the migraine threshold, so patients can tolerate more triggers before getting a headache.

The mechanism of how this raising of the threshold happens is currently unknown. There are several of these medications. The first are a class of medicines called Tricyclic Antidepressants. These include medicines like nortriptyline and amitriptyline. These medications were originally developed to treat depression, but can be used to prevent migraines as well (as well as other conditions like nerve pain or chronic cough). When I am prescribing anti-migraine medications, I typically start with a tricyclic antidepressant for a few reasons. They are usually well tolerated with low side effects, they are only once-a-day dosing (at bedtime), and they are usually inexpensive.

There are also anti-seizure medications that are used for the purposes of migraine prevention. These include medicines like Topamax and Depakote. In my experience, these medicines can help but tend to have more side effects and sometimes more frequent dosing schedules.

Finally, there are several different medicines that were originally used to treat high blood pressure that can be used to prevent migraines. These include beta blocker medications as well as other drugs called calcium channel blockers. I generally use these as a last resort because there is a risk of lowering the blood pressure too much, especially if my patient is already on other blood pressure medicines.

As an aside, I much more commonly prescribe preventive migraine medications for the treatment of migraine-associated dizziness (which can occur even in the absence of headaches). For difficult-to-treat headaches (especially those that do not respond to the RESET treatment), I will usually defer to the patient's neurologist for adjusting and trying these various medications.

What is the one, two, three system?

This is a system described in the book I mentioned earlier, Heal Your Headache. The 1-2-3 system can potentially be used to eliminate or lower the number of migraine headaches. Like the name says, there are three steps in the system.

Step one is to eliminate all abortive medications including the triptans, opioids or Fioricet. Typically, this will take several weeks to several months to get completely out of someone's system. During this time, there is the possibility that the headaches can temporarily get much worse as patients withdraw and rebound from their overuse of abortive medicines.

Step two is to eliminate migraine triggers. Usually, this will require a significant amount of detective work by the patient. They'll need to radically cleanse their diet for at least a few weeks, if not a few months. Over time, people can start reintroducing foods and see what foods cause headache symptoms and which ones are okay.

Patients will need to really work on getting good quality sleep (7-8 hours or more <u>every night</u>) and doing everything else possible to eliminate and identify triggers.

Step 3 in the 1-2-3 system will only be necessary for some people. If step one and two do not get rid of the migraines completely, then patients move on to step three and in that case, they would add one or more preventive medications. Dr. Buchholz, the author of this system, claims that it will basically eliminate migraines for just about anyone.

What are other medical options?

Other options that neurologists or pain medicine specialists offer include Botox injections for migraines. Botox is actually a deadly poison in large amounts, but when used in an appropriately low amount, can cause temporary muscle paralysis where it is injected. There are a number of medical functions it is used for: the most well-known being for smoothing of wrinkles on the face.

For migraine prevention, Botox is usually injected in certain areas around the forehead and scalp. By blocking muscle function in these areas, the treatment can potentially lower the numbers of migraines. It is not entirely clear how this works, but most likely the muscle relaxation helps to lower the inflammation in the muscles due to the migraine mechanism.

A large study called PREEMPT showed that patients with chronic migraine who had Botox injections done every 12 weeks had 8-9 fewer headache days per month than their pre-treatment baseline. However, patients in the study who were injected with placebo (saline solution with no Botox in it) also experienced improvement of 6-7 fewer headache days per month.

Another medical treatment that can potentially be used in very severe chronic migraine cases is IV infusion of ketamine. Ketamine is a powerful psychedelic drug, which is used in anesthesia and in other hospital settings. In very severe migraines, this can sometimes work to eliminate the headaches.

What are dietary triggers?

The number one dietary trigger by far is caffeine. This makes sense if you think about it. One of the major effects of caffeine is to cause constriction of blood vessels. As a result, this can block migraines, but when the caffeine wears off, the migraine will frequently come roaring back. This is a massive setup for a vicious cycle of caffeine overuse with awful rebound headaches. If you had to eliminate only one thing to help your migraines, avoiding caffeine would be it.

There are a huge potential number of other dietary triggers. These include monosodium glutamate (MSG), chocolate, alcoholic beverages (especially red wine), nuts, processed meats, cheese (especially aged cheese), and citrus. In truth, basically anything can be a dietary trigger for you because of the large variability among different people. Really, the only way to determine your own triggers are to eliminate almost everything and then start experimenting and seeing if certain foods and beverages cause headache symptoms or not.

What are unavoidable or hard to avoid triggers?

The first of these is weather or barometric pressure changes. This could be from storms, cold fronts, heat or humidity, air travel, or changes in altitude. Next would be hormonal changes. As discussed above, these are most common in women including menstruation, pregnancy or menopause. Potentially, hormonal changes in men can also be a trigger.

The next hard-to-avoid trigger is various chemicals or sensory stimuli such as perfume, smoke, cleaning products or bright light. Physical exertion can also be a trigger of migraines. This includes bending over, cardio exercise, weight lifting, sex, or dehydration. Again, as mentioned before, sleep deprivation and stress are huge triggers of migraines.

What are non-medical treatments for migraines?

There are a number of options for migraine treatment and prevention that do not involve taking any medication. The first I'll discuss is called biofeedback. This is a method that can be used to control the headaches by controlling your body through deep breathing and mental focus. Many times, patients are able to learn how to lower or raise their heart rate by controlling their breath. By doing this, they can actually relax and have improvement in their migraine headaches from stress reduction. There are various resources online and then also training practitioners that can teach people how to do biofeedback. My impression is that it can be helpful in some people but not effective in others, and that it takes a fair amount of practice to get good at it.

The next treatment is not really a treatment at all, it is more of a lifestyle change. This "treatment" is to consistently sleep at least seven to eight hours per night. Sleeping well can sometimes be hard especially if patients have small children to take care of (myself at the time of writing this book!) or are working long hours. But without adequate sleep, the risk of migraines is much higher.

Yoga can be a very helpful way to treat migraines. Yoga is very relaxing and is also a form of exercise. Both its stress-relief and its exercise aspects can help to lower the number of migraines. Exercising for 30 minutes at least five days a week has also been shown to help with lowering the numbers and intensity of migraines. For busy people, though, it is easier said than done to carve out enough time to exercise 5 days a week.

Next, acupuncture is a way to potentially treat migraines. Acupuncture was originally developed in Asia and involves placing very tiny needles at various pressure points and energy points throughout the body. People who are trained in acupuncture can identify different parts of the body that contribute to migraines and can try and stimulate those areas to lower the headaches. Acupuncture is typically covered by insurance as well.

Finally, there is a non-invasive medical device called Cefaly (cefaly.us) which is placed onto the forehead. This device delivers a low level electrical stimulation to the forehead that stimulates the trigeminal nerve. It can be used daily (for 20 minutes at a time) to help prevent headaches or used on an as-needed basis to treat active headaches (60 minute treatment).

What is my opinion of all of these treatments?

I think there are a lot of different options for people with migraines. There are many more options than I think most people realize. However, sometimes having too many options is almost worse than having not enough options. Think back to the Las Vegas buffet analogy: when there are 100 things on the menu, it is hard to figure out what to eat! It can be very confusing and very hard to decide what kind of treatments to try. The other thing that makes this all confusing and difficult is that the most effective treatment (or combination of treatments) will vary widely for different individuals. What may help dramatically for one person may do nothing or even make the headache worse for another person.

Almost all of the time, there's going to be some experimenting and trying different things before a particular person finds the right treatment for themself. As a general rule, I have come to this conclusion after my research about the "State of the Art" treatment for migraine: getting good control of your migraines will require a major lifestyle change and significant diligence and willpower. It will also take a large amount of your time. Sometimes patients may need to temporarily get worse before getting better with the state-of-the-art migraine treatments. I can certainly see how all these possibilities and options are intimidating for many migraineurs. As a result, it's potentially easier just to keep taking over-the-counter medicines and live with it.

What if there was a better way to treat migraines? Perhaps a simple office treatment without any significant side effects and with a minimal time commitment? In part one of this book, we've covered what's typically done for migraines for most people and we're now going to move on to part two, where I discuss this new option, the RESET treatment.

Seth H. Evans, M.D.

Chapter 5:

Target the Source

Seth H. Evans, M.D.

5 TARGET THE SOURCE

Wait a minute! I just said we were about to discuss the RESET treatment. Why am I now starting to babble in medical jargon? What is this sphenopalatine mumbo-jumbo?

Well, the reason I've thrown out this curveball is that the RESET treatment and the sphenopalatine ganglion block are two names for the same thing. However, the RESET treatment is a specific way I have developed to perform a sphenopalatine ganglion block. You'll be an expert on all this in a few more pages, I promise! For now, let's get started with the basics and we will build your knowledge from there.

What is a brief definition of sphenopalatine ganglion block?

Sphenopalatine ganglion block is a pretty long and intimidating name for what is actually a simple treatment. Going forward, I'll frequently abbreviate it to SPG block so I can avoid getting carpal tunnel syndrome from typing that long name out over and over!

First, let's break up the name into its three different words.

Starting with the final word "<u>block</u>", this treatment is a nerve block. If you've ever had dental work done, you have personally experienced a nerve block. This occurred when your dentist injected novacaine or lidocaine into your mouth to numb your teeth. Likewise, during the SPG block, we are blocking a nerve called the Sphenopalatine Ganglion. Instead of in the back of your mouth where your dentist injects, the SPG is in inside of your nose in the very back.

What is the sphenopalatine ganglion (SPG)?

<u>Sphenopalatine</u> refers to the location of the nerve. Although I usually refer to the SPG as a single entity throughout this book, there are actually two of them, one inside each side of your nose. Each sphenopalatine ganglion has the exact same function for the half of your head that it lives in.

Many people don't realize that the skull is not just one bone. It's actually made up of a number of different bones that are fused together during development and in the first years of life. Two of those bones are called the sphenoid bone and the palatine bone. Near where these two bone are fused in the middle of the head is this little nerve bundle called the sphenopalatine ganglion.

A nerve bundle is what the word ganglion means. It's an area on the nerve that appears to be swollen or enlarged. In this bulge on the nerve is where the cell bodies of the millions of neurons that compose the nerve live. Outward from these cell bodies extend long fibers called axons that transmit electrical signals back and forth from the brain to the surrounding tissues. These long axons make up most of the length of our nerves.

The sphenopalatine ganglion itself contains three different types of nerve fibers. The first of those is what are called somatosensory fibers. These are nerves that carry sensations from the head and the face back to the brain. If you tap your finger on your cheek, the electrical signals that relay sensation of that tapping will actually travel through the sphenopalatine ganglion on their way back to your brain.

There are also two other types of nerve fibers that travel from the brain through the SPG out to the surrounding tissues of the head and the face. These are both types of autonomic nerve fibers. Autonomic means that these nerves communicate functions that happen without your conscious control. These functions include many different things, such as sweating, salivation, or digestion.

The two types of autonomic fibers are called sympathetic and parasympathetic. Typically, sympathetic nerve signals trigger what we call the "fight or flight response," when your adrenalin gets up. The parasympathetic fibers cause "rest and digest" functions. There are many other functions that these nerve fibers control, but that is a topic beyond the scope of this book.

In the head and the neck, these two different autonomic fibers control the production of saliva or mucus in the nose, as well as sweating, tearing, and other unconscious processes.

In essence, the sphenopalatine ganglion is a relay center. Autonomic signals are transmitted from the brain out to the head/face and sensory signals are picked up out in the head and face and are sent back to the brain through the SPG.

Additionally, the sphenopalatine ganglion is located on one of the major branches of the trigeminal nerve. If you remember back to Chapter One, you may remember the important role that the trigeminal nerve plays in migraine headaches. This nerve provides sensation to most of the head including the lining around the brain (known as the meninges). It's the main nerve that mediates migraine headaches.

To get an idea of the power of the SPG, think about what would happen if you ate a large scoop of ice cream as fast as you can. Yes, that cold ice cream going in your mouth all at once will cause you to get a sudden severe stabbing pain. I've always called it "brain freeze," but sometimes it's called ice cream headache. This severe pain is due to stimulation of the SPG by the sudden temperature change. Fortunately, when you stop eating the ice cream, the tissue warms back up quickly and the brain freeze goes away.

The SPG is a direct connection to the brain. It's literally right underneath the brain. By blocking this area, we can trigger a beneficial effect on the processes within your brain that are triggering the migraine headaches.

Where is the sphenopalatine ganglion?

The SPG is in the very back of your nasal cavity, right underneath the thin lining known as the mucosa. This location is important for a couple of reasons. Number one, the SPG is pretty easily accessible for treatment or intervention. The reason is that it's the only place in your whole body where a nerve that contains both types of autonomic fibers and somatosensory fibers is so close to the outside world. It may not seem like way back inside your nose is close to the outside world, but any air-filled space is considered "outside the body," even though it is technically inside your nose.

Typically, the sphenopalatine ganglion is between one and five millimeters under the mucosal lining in the nose. This is not just trivia! Because the ganglion is so close under the lining, it is possible for me to squirt numbing medication over the proper area, and that medication can diffuse into the ganglion and block it without the need for needle injection.

What is the sphenopalatine ganglion's role in migraines?

Once again, the ganglion is located directly on one of the major branches of the trigeminal nerve. During migraines, there are chaotic signals traveling up and down this nerve that cause pain sensation to be transferred up to the brain and instructions for dilation of blood vessels and inflammation to travel out to the peripheral head and face.

By this two-way signal pathway, there can be chronic dysregulation of blood flow through the head and the neck that can cause chronic migraines. These nerve processes are not well understood, but this is the summary of the most current research in these areas.

What does a nerve block mean?

It means just what it sounds like! A doctor can use local anesthetic like lidocaine to temporarily block the function of any nerve. By using this medication, the signals that are traveling to and from the brain are temporarily blocked and cannot transmit through the nerve.

In order to block a nerve, it is obviously necessary to place the local anesthetic in the same location as the nerve. Most of the time, this is done through needle injection. Again, if you've ever been to the dentist, you know what this is like (it's not super fun). Sometimes, though, it's possible for the medication to get in to the nerve through diffusion. So we can just place the medicine topically and allow it to transmit into the nerve that way. Fortunately, this is easily achievable to block the SPG.

What happens when the sphenopalatine ganglion is blocked?

Temporarily, there will be a loss of function through that branch of the trigeminal nerve. The amount of time depends on the type of local anesthetic that is used to block the nerve. In the case of lidocaine (the medication I use), the blocking effect normally lasts for 2-3 hours.

When the SPG is blocked, you will probably feel some decreased sensation in your face, usually over the cheek below the eyes. There can also be a temporary decrease in nasal congestion and runny nose due to the autonomic fibers traveling through the ganglion. There can also be warming of the skin of your cheek.

All of these effects are interesting, but let's get to the real benefit of blocking the SPG (the reason you're reading this book!). By blocking the ganglion, we can potentially stop a migraine headache as well as prevent headaches in the future for some amount of time.

Once the nerve block wears off in a few hours, the normal sensation and autonomic function will be restored. However, the improvement in migraines typically lasts for some time longer.

How does this happen? Well, unfortunately I don't have a great answer for you. The mechanism is still poorly understood. We do know that by blocking the sphenopalatine ganglion, there is a release of a chemical called Nitric Oxide inside your brain. This chemical trigger causes deep muscle relaxation and can actually allow healing and pain relief throughout the body.

Because of this nitric oxide release, the SPG block can also potentially help other medical problems including neck or back pain. However, these alternative treatments are out of the scope of this book (perhaps they will be discussed further in a future book!).

What are the results of SPG block as a treatment for migraines?

First of all, every patient is going to be different. Some people respond amazingly and others will have no improvement at all. Based on the research that's been done over the years on this treatment, I expect that 80% to 90% of patients with migraines will have some amount of benefit for some amount of time after having the treatment. About 68% of patients who receive a SPG block will still have some improvement in their headaches one month after they've had the treatment.

This does not necessarily mean that 68% will have zero headaches for a month afterward. It means that 68% of people will still be at least a little better 1 month later than before having the SPG block. For a few lucky folks, the effects of the treatment could even last for several months. Patients who suffer from more severe or more frequent migraines will probably have a shorter duration of benefit.

Can the SPG block be repeated?

Yes! In fact, you can safely receive this treatment as often as every day. The good news is that there is really no downside or increased risk to having repeated SPG blocks. Specifically, there is no risk of rebound headache with this treatment as opposed to many other migraine treatments we discussed in earlier chapters.

Can sphenopalatine ganglion block be used for other conditions than migraine?

Yes. Again, the focus of this book is on the treatment and prevention of migraines. I will direct readers to the references section at the end of this book for a list of conditions that may be helped by the SPG block. Readers should be aware that SPG block is usually not covered by insurance for treatment of conditions outside of the head (such as back pain or sciatica).

We'll now move onto the next chapter, where you'll learn all about the history of the SPG block and the various ways it has been performed over the years.

Seth H. Evans, M.D.

Chapter 6:

Know the Past to Know the Present

Seth H. Evans, M.D.

6 KNOW THE PAST TO KNOW THE PRESENT

If you've made it this far into the book, I couldn't blame you if you assumed that the SPG block is some sort of brand-new cutting edge therapy. It's pretty amazing that in the several books I read during my research of "state of the art" treatment of migraines, I literally found zero mention of the SPG block anywhere! But far from being a brand new treatment, the SPG block has actually been around for over 100 years!

When was the SPG block first done?

Originally, the sphenopalatine ganglion block was performed and described in the medical literature in 1909 by Dr. Greenfield Sluder. Dr. Sluder was an ENT specialist at Washington University in St. Louis. He had a particular interest in the treatment of headaches and facial pain syndromes. In fact, there remains to this day a disorder called Sluder's Neuralgia. Over the years, this term has become used for a few different problems. But initially, it meant a facial headache. Dr. Sluder originally started performing the SPG block in order to treat migraines and other types of facial pain syndromes.

Once he started publishing his good results in the ENT literature, some of his colleagues throughout the country started trying the treatment as well.

How has the sphenopalatine ganglion block developed since then?

So, back in the early 20th century, ENT doctors like myself were the ones performing the SPG block. One of these doctors has been profiled in a book called *Miracles on Park Avenue* by Albert Gerber. His name was Dr. Milton Reder, and he practiced in Manhattan for almost 70 years starting in the 1920s up until his death in the 1980s. Dr. Reder initially practiced the entire spectrum of the ear, nose and throat specialty, but later transitioned his practice to exclusively performing the SPG block. He would often perform the treatment over 100 times a day in his clinic, 7 days a week!

Dr. Reder was able to get amazing results for not just migraine headaches, but for many other medical conditions including chronic back pain, sciatica, and a wide variety of other diseases. The book *Miracles on Park Avenue* provides numerous fascinating stories of different patients who had amazing recoveries under his care after months or years of suffering. Sadly, Dr. Reder was ostracized by the medical establishment in

New York because of his unorthodox ways, but at the same time, many doctors secretly sent him patients when they had run out of "mainstream" options to offer.

Dr. Reder treated numerous celebrities and prominent people including the actor, Yul Brynner, who played the King in the film, *The King and I*. Much more about this fascinating story can be found in the book *Miracles on Park Avenue* by Albert Gerber. The book is out of print, but used copies can be found for sale on Amazon and other places online.

What has been the history of the sphenopalatine ganglion block in the past few decades?

Over time, the SPG block gradually migrated away from ear, nose and throat doctors to other specialists who more commonly treated headaches and facial pain. These specialists were typically neurologists and pain medicine specialists. Eventually, it became a forgotten treatment among ear, nose and throat specialists. I know that I never heard anything about the SPG block in my training.

Ultimately, we have ended up in a strange situation. We know that the sphenopalatine ganglion is inside the nose. And who are the experts at working inside the nose? Well, ear, nose and throat doctors, of course.

The problem is that neurologists are generally the doctors who are treating migraines and other types of headaches. Neurologists are not trained in how to examine the nasal cavity or perform any nasal procedures.

Pain medicine doctors are the experts in nerve blocks throughout other parts of the body, but they're used to injecting medication with needles and using x-rays for proper placement of the needle. Most pain medicine procedures are done in the operating room under anesthesia.

We're now in a situation where this amazing treatment for migraines is not well known by the doctors treating migraines (neurologists). And the doctors best suited to perform this treatment (ENT doctors), are really not aware of the SPG block at all.

How has the sphenopalatine ganglion block traditionally been performed?

For most of the history of the SPG block, there have been two methods. The most common method is called intranasal. Traditionally (and still by many doctors today), intranasal SPG block was performed by placing a long Q-tip or a wire applicator with cotton on the end. The cotton tip is blindly placed by the doctor into the back of the nasal cavity. Prior to being placed, the end of the Q-tip is soaked with a local anesthetic, usually either cocaine or lidocaine.

The doctor placing the Q-tip is able to look in the front of the nose, but it is almost never possible to see all the way back to where the SPG is located. As a result, the Q-tip is placed blindly towards the back of the nose in the general direction of the SPG. After it is placed, the Q-tip needs to sit in place for 30 minutes before being removed. This allows time for the local anesthetic to diffuse from the cotton tip through the mucosal lining into the SPG. In the book I mentioned earlier, there are a number of amusing stories about Dr. Reder's waiting room full of people with long wires sticking out of their nose.

The second common way that the sphenopalatine ganglion block has been performed in recent years is called transfacial. This method is (to my knowledge) only performed by pain medicine specialists. It is done using X-ray guidance to place a needle through the skin of the face all the way down to where the ganglion is located. Once the needle is properly placed on the x-ray, local anesthetic is injected around the SPG. If SPG block is performed transfacially, it needs to be done in the operating room under sedation. It is a technically challenging procedure to perform and normally takes between 30 and 60 minutes from start to finish.

Why has intranasal sphenopalatine ganglion block always been done blindly?

When the SPG block was first developed in 1909, there was no such thing as a nasal endoscope. At this time, ear, nose and throat doctors were mainly the physicians doing this treatment, but they didn't have the tools that we now have, so they would just look in the front of the nose and place the Q-tip blindly back to where the ganglion is located.

In more recent times, any doctors who are doing this treatment are not typically ENT doctors and they are not trained in our modern methods of nasal endoscopy. As a result, most are still using the old-fashioned blind placement of Q-tips. This includes the large majority of current physicians and dentists who offer the SPG block. In addition, some pain medicine specialists offer the treatment via the transfacial needle injection route.

Are there new techniques for performing blind intranasal SPG block?

Yes. There are actually three medical devices on the market now that can be used to blindly perform this treatment in the nose. The first of those is called the SphenoCath. The SphenoCath has a special place in my heart because if not for it, I would never have learned about the SPG block at all. I received some promotional material about this device in 2016 which started my journey researching the SPG block treatment.

The SphenoCath is a disposable medical device that is angled in such a way that it can spray lidocaine into the back of the nasal cavity to reliably perform SPG block. There's also a device called the Allevio, which is very similar to the SphenoCath. Both of these devices have a thin catheter that's placed blindly into the nose and tend to inject the local anesthetic in roughly the correct place.

The third device is called the Tx360. It is stuck blindly into the back of the nose and has an angled injector, which sprays the local anesthetic near the area of the sphenopalatine ganglion. All of these methods spray the medicine. There's no needle sticks with any of them.

Overall, my opinion is that these 3 devices are all reasonable options if you can't see inside the nose and are thus forced to perform the SPG block blindly. Most of the time, I feel it would be easier for a doctor to get the local anesthetic to the right spot using one of these devices than trying to place a q-tip.

Why has the sphenopalatine ganglion block never caught on?

I think there are several reasons. The traditional intranasal method of performing the treatment is technically challenging and quite delicate if you want to do it without scraping the inside of the nose or causing a lot of discomfort. The doctors who are normally treating migraine are not the doctors who are experts in nasal anatomy and endoscopy of the nose.

As a result, I think the SPG block can be very intimidating for neurologists or other non-ENT doctors to perform. As an ENT specialist, I see a lot of patients with anatomic problems like deviated septum or swollen tissues in the nose that would make blind placement of a q-tip into the posterior nasal cavity difficult or impossible. I would not be surprised if many non-ENT specialists who try to perform the SPG block are wary of trying it again due to an unpleasant experience.

In addition, it has never been conventional wisdom or "mainstream therapy" over the years to try this treatment. Usually, doctors want to prescribe medications. Most of us docs are not necessarily trying to learn a new and unfamiliar procedure, especially non-surgeons. There are also no drug reps pushing this treatment, but there are plenty of them pushing the latest and greatest triptan or other medication for migraines. For many physicians, it's easier to just write a prescription for a triptan than trying to learn an unfamiliar procedure.

Finally, ENT doctors generally don't treat migraines, though we do see it all the time. As a result, the sphenopalatine ganglion block treatment has been somewhat lost to the general knowledge of ear, nose and throat doctors until the recent times.

Chapter 7:

Migraine RESET

7 MIGRAINE RESET

So now we have finally made it to (in my humble opinion) the most important part of the book. Give yourself a pat on the back for reading this far!

When I first learned of the SPG block a couple years ago and began researching it more and more, I was really struck by the paradox of it. Here was this 100+ year old treatment that was at the same time a revolutionary advance in the treatment of migraine headaches and many other problems. My mind quickly started brainstorming how I could implement this amazing treatment in my own practice. This chapter will give you all the details on the method I've developed and why I think it is substantially better than the alternatives of the past 100 years.

What is my method for performing sphenopalatine ganglion block?

I call my method the RESET Treatment. RESET stands for **R**elieve and **E**liminate **S**ymptoms **E**ndoscopic **T**reatment. I decided to rename my method of SPG block for a few reasons. First, the term RESET is a good summary of the outcome of having the treatment. It really is like "hitting the reset button" on your headaches or other symptoms.

Let's break down the abbreviation RESET: having this treatment can both **R**elieve the **S**ymptoms of headache you're currently feeling and **E**liminate headaches for some time in the future. **E**ndoscopic **T**reatment refers to the fact that I use a thin endoscope to see inside the nose to accurately and reliably place the local anesthetic onto the SPG (more on this below). Finally, RESET is just easier to say and remember. "Endoscopic sphenopalatine ganglion block" does not exactly roll off your tongue very easily.

My method is as follows: First, I will use Afrin spray to decongest the inside of your nose. Ideally, the Afrin is sprayed into both sides of your nose at least 10 minutes before performing the RESET treatment. Afrin is available over the counter without a prescription, so you can actually spray it in your nose at home before coming in to my office. By decongesting your nose first, it will allow me much more room to maneuver and to see far back into the nose where the SPG is located.

Second, I'll use a nasal endoscope to look into your nose while I perform the treatment. The great benefit of the endoscope is that I can actually see what I'm doing! (Shocking, eh?) For over 100 years, almost every SPG block has been done blindly either by shoving Q-tips in the nose or by injecting through the face with a needle. Trust me: it's a lot easier to perform this treatment when you can see what you're doing. The use of a nasal endoscope is really where the RESET treatment stands above and beyond any traditional method of performing SPG block.

So now I can see into the back of your nose with my endoscope. What local anesthetic do I use and how do I get it into the right spot? I use 1 milliliter of 2% lidocaine on each side of your nose, and I inject this using a syringe and a thin blunt catheter (i.e. no needles).

During the injection of the lidocaine, you will be lying on your back with your neck extended (with your chin up). This positioning of your head allows the lidocaine to pool directly over the sphenopalatine ganglion, so that it can diffuse in and take effect. The entire injection part of the RESET treatment for both sides of your nose takes me less than one minute and usually is even less than 30 seconds to perform. It is not painful. The first time you have the treatment, it will feel weird and uncomfortable. You will be feeling strange sensations in places where you're not used to feeling them, but it's usually not painful other than maybe a brief stinging (like when you accidentally inhale water in your nose while swimming). After a treatment or two, it is generally no big deal, especially once you start seeing the improvement in your headaches.

The RESET treatment does not require any sedation. Obviously, the treatment is done in my office, not in an operating room. After the treatment, I will have you lie on your back with head extended for 5 to 10 minutes to allow the lidocaine to diffuse into the ganglion.

Why is RESET better?

First of all, I can see what I'm doing. Using the endoscope allows me to reliably place the local anesthetic over the SPG. The analogy I like to use is if you had to press a button, would you rather have it right in front of you or try and reach behind your back blindly to press the button? Obviously, anything is easier to do when you can see what you're doing!

As an ENT specialist, I'm an expert in the anatomy of the nose and I'm very used to working inside of the noses of awake patients with an endoscope. I know how to do this safely and with minimal discomfort for my patients. In fact, normally I'm doing things in people's noses that are potentially a lot more uncomfortable than the RESET treatment (such as sinus procedures or removing nasal polyps). Now, any other ear, nose and throat doctor can say the same, but neurologists and pain medicine doctors are not trained in doing these things.

Finally, with the positioning I use for the treatment (lying on your back with chin up), I'm able to use gravity to my advantage to keep the lidocaine pooled in the perfect position around the sphenopalatine ganglion. The alternative would be the old-fashioned Q-tip method, where the cotton tip needs to be placed perfectly and sit there for 30 minutes to have a good effect. If the end of the q-tip shifts or is not placed precisely to begin with, it won't work.

How often should patients have the RESET treatment?

There are no official guidelines for this. For every individual patient, I have certain goals in the short term (the first few weeks of treatments) and in the long term. My ultimate goal is to get the best possible result for you with the lowest frequency of treatments in the long term.

However, when we first start your RESET treatments, the goal is different. At that point, my goal is to see:
1. If the treatment works for you at all
2. If it does work, what is the maximum benefit you can get from the treatment

So, what I do currently for new patients (February 2018) is to perform the RESET treatment once and then see you back in a week. By that time, you will have either noticed some benefit or not. If there was zero improvement in your headaches, the RESET treatment is likely not effective for you.

If you did have some improvement in your migraines, I would then recommend that you have the RESET treatment as often as possible for one week. Ideally, this would be every day (Mon-Fri) for 1 week. After that, we can usually space the treatments out to twice a week for a few weeks and then to once a week and so on, depending on how you do. If you start getting headaches (or have a worsening in your headaches), we know that we spaced the treatments too infrequently and we should probably do them more often.

Here's an example of a patient I'm currently treating for chronic migraines. She is a very nice lady in her 60s and had been suffering from migraines 2-3 times a week for years. After her first RESET treatment, she noticed a dramatic improvement in her headaches for several days. As a result, she underwent daily treatments for one week and had no headaches at all during that time. Over the next few months, we gradually spaced out her treatments and she continued to have zero headaches.

Eventually, she went 1 month between RESET treatments, but she had a migraine during the last week before her next scheduled treatment. From this information, we were able to deduce that every 3 week treatments was the optimal frequency for her. She has now been receiving every 3 week treatments for several months with zero headaches. She is one of the the happiest people I get to see in this job!

If you come in for migraines and decide to try the RESET treatment, your results may be different. You potentially could have complete elimination of headaches but require more frequent treatments. Or you could still get the same number of headaches but each one is 50% milder than before. Or you could have half as many headaches but they are just as bad as before. Ultimately, it's up to you to decide if the benefit of the treatments is worth the cost in money and time.

What are the risks or downsides of the treatment?

As a doctor and a surgeon, I am very used to listing the risks and possible complications of medical procedures. The RESET treatment is literally the least risky thing that I offer in my practice. It has zero risk of any life-threatening or permanent complication. There is a low risk of mild and temporary unpleasant side effects.

During the 30-60 seconds it takes me to perform the RESET treatment, there is usually some brief mild discomfort, which can sometimes seem worse for patients who are very anxious. Usually, after one or two treatments, patients know what to expect and there's much less anxiety. It's not unusual that people can be nervous the first time because the treatment is unknown.

Some of the lidocaine usually ends up dripping into the throat. So, there may be a bad taste in the mouth and a temporary numb feeling in the throat, which usually wears off in about one hour. There may also be a brief burning sensation when the lidocaine is squirted into the nose. This usually lasts for less than one minute. There's an extremely low risk of a minor nose bleed, but normally, since I can see what I'm doing, I'm not scraping anything in the nose.

Rarely, patients may have what's called a vasovagal response. This is a reflex response that can occur when the inside of someone's nose is manipulated (or for many other reasons). If you've ever gotten lightheaded or passed out at the sight of blood or because you forgot to eat breakfast, you've had a vasovagal response. People feel lightheaded, cold and clammy and potentially feel nauseated. At worst, some people may faint briefly. Usually, the vasovagal reflex will wear off in a few minutes and it's not typically dangerous.

Very rarely, there can be a temporary increase in the severity of the headache or dizziness. I have not seen either of these complications in my practice. Fortunately, there are no serious risks to the RESET treatment. There is zero chance that it could cause death, a serious medical issue, or any kind of permanent complication.

Who should have the RESET treatment?

For the purposes of this book, anyone who has frequent bothersome migraine headaches. How often is frequent and how bad is bothersome is up to each individual. In addition, patients with other types of headaches or facial pain syndromes can also potentially benefit from the RESET treatment. Patients with TMJ pain can also get some help and relief.

There are also many other types of pain including back and neck pain, and sciatica that can also be improved with the RESET treatment. This improvement in outside of the head conditions is thought to be caused by modulatory effects on nitric oxide pathways in the brain through signaling from the sphenopalatine ganglion. Ultimately, patients need to weigh benefits of the treatment versus the risk. The RESET treatment, as I said before, has essentially no serious risks. I'm really willing to try it on almost anyone. If it doesn't work, it doesn't work. But, there's no harm and no foul in trying.

Who cannot have the RESET treatment?

Anyone with an anatomic problem in the nose where I can't get the scope in or get the medicine in cannot have the procedure unless the anatomic problem is fixed. This would include people with severely deviated septums or with large nasal polyps. In addition, some patients with severe sinus infections may not be able to have the procedure due to swelling and congestion. If these anatomic issues are addressed with medication or surgical procedures, the RESET treatment can be done at that point.

If a patient has extremely severe congestion in the nose that will not open up with decongestants, we may not be able to do the RESET treatment. If a patient previously had sinus surgery, it is possible that the RESET treatment won't work due to scar tissue blocking diffusion of the lidocaine to the SPG, but we can usually still try it in these cases- the worst case scenario is the treatment won't help.

Finally, if a patient is allergic to either lidocaine or Afrin, which are the 2 medications used, they should not have the treatment. We could conceivably try a different medication such as bupivacaine or another local anesthetic, but I've not had to deal with that in my practice so far.

What is my philosophy on the RESET treatment?

My goal is to quickly identify who responds to the RESET treatment and who doesn't. If you have the treatment and your headaches don't get any better, I don't want you to have to pay for it. I don't like to charge money for something that doesn't work. If you go a week after your first treatment and there's been no improvement in your headaches, I will not bill for the procedure.

For the majority of patients who do respond to the RESET treatment, I recommend to do it frequently at first. As I said before, everyday for a week is usually the best way to start doing these treatments. At that point, we'll space things out until we find the right balance of symptom control versus the time and cost for every individual. My goal is to make it easy for you to come in to my office as much or as little as you want to achieve your personal goal of headache control.

Chapter 8:

Frequently Asked Questions

Seth H. Evans, M.D.

8 FREQUENTLY ASKED QUESTIONS

Am I a candidate for the RESET treatment?

Yes. If you have bothersome migraine headaches, you should certainly consider trying this treatment. RESET may also help you if you have any other type of headache, facial pain syndrome, or temporomandibular joint pain. For pain conditions within the head, the RESET treatment is usually covered by insurance. Patients with chronic neck or back pain, sciatica, or a number of other conditions can be helped by the RESET treatment as well. Unfortunately, the treatment is generally not covered by insurance for problems in the neck or below the neck. I do offer a cash pay price or financing options for those with no insurance or if your insurance does not approve the treatment. If the RESET works to relieve your pain, it may be worth whatever cost you might pay.

Is there a difference between a sphenopalatine ganglion block and the RESET treatment?

RESET is the name I call my particular method of performing the sphenopalatine ganglion block. So, all RESET treatments are also SPG blocks. However, there are other ways to perform sphenopalatine block, such as the intranasal q-tip method or the transfacial needle injection method. These other methods of SPG block are not the same as the RESET treatment.

Can I do other migraine treatments at the same time?

Yes. There's no reason you can't do any other treatment including medications, diet changes, lowering other triggers, and/or any kind of complementary or alternative treatments. I do not want anyone to stop doing any other helpful treatment just because they are having the RESET treatment. Although sometimes the RESET treatments alone are the answer to your migraine problem, they can also serve as a complementary treatment to anything else that you might be doing.

What if my primary care doctor or my neurologist discourages me from having the RESET treatment?

First of all, the most likely reason they would discourage you is because they don't know about the RESET treatment at all. Even if they have heard of the SPG block, they don't know the specific way that I have developed to perform this treatment. If your doctor does know anything about the SPG block as it's traditionally been done, they might think that I'm going to put you under anesthesia in the operating room. They may also think that I'm trying to do the old-fashioned Q-tip method. If your neurologist has ever tried to do a SPG block, they may have had a bad experience with it due to their lack of training in nasal procedures.

As a general rule, I have found that many doctors are very conservative and they reflexively recommend against anything that's not "mainstream," "conventionally done," or "evidence-based". Frequently, this includes anything that they've never personally heard of. As a result, you may run into some resistance if you bring this up with your regular doctor or neurologist. My opinion is that there's so little risk to having the RESET treatment and such a high potential benefit that it's worth your time to try it no matter what your regular doctor says. The worst possible outcome is that it doesn't help you, and even then you haven't lost anything. It will not make any other medical condition worse, and it will not limit any other options that you might consider for treating your migraines or other chronic pain condition.

Should I continue seeing my neurologist, pain medicine specialist, or primary care doctor, etc?

Yes. I offer the RESET treatment as one part of a global approach to treating migraine. I strongly encourage all of my patients to keep their regular follow-up with their headache specialist and their other doctors. Though a lot of my patients may get complete relief from regular RESET treatments alone, many of them will still need other medical treatments or non-medical interventions to adequately control their migraines. I don't want you to lose out on these benefits and focus exclusively on what I do. Migraine is a bad problem, and you should do everything you can to get the most possible relief from your headaches.

What if I had the sphenopalatine ganglion block before and it didn't work?

It really depends on the method of the treatment that you had before and who was performing it. The q-tip intranasal method is not reliable if the medication-soaked tip is not precisely placed. This misplacement is more likely in non-experienced hands. In my practice as an ENT, I spend a lot of time working inside people's noses. I can safely say that reliably and precisely putting a Q-tip into the exact right spot in the back of the nose is no easy feat, particularly if you're placing it blindly.

Of course there are experts like Dr. Milton Reder, who probably performed over a million of these treatments during his 60 years of practice in New York City. Absolutely, he could do it and do it reliably. But if the SPG block is not something that's performed routinely by your doctor, they may not know how to do it right and their technique may not be reliable.

I will tell you for certain, my way of doing this treatment is different than whatever you might have had before. It is simple for me to do this. I perform nasal endoscopy many times every day in my clinic, whether it's for migraine treatments or for other more complicated procedures in the nose. I know how to keep patients comfortable while I'm working in their noses, and I am 100% confident I can perform the RESET treatment reliably. So, it is probably a good idea for you to try the RESET treatment, even if you've previously failed to respond after a traditional SPG block.

What if my doctor wants to perform the sphenopalatine ganglion block on me?

It is obviously your personal decision as to who does what to your own body. So, of course it is fine if you want to have another doctor do your SPG block.. If you're considering having another practitioner perform this treatment, I would recommend that you ask them how they will perform it and how often they have done it in the past. Almost certainly, you will be getting a traditional SPG block, not the RESET method that I have developed. The advantages of my practice are the accuracy and reliable placement of the lidocaine and the convenience and efficiency that I am able to create for people coming in to have this treatment.

Are there any restrictions after the RESET treatment?

Yes, there are several. First of all, it's advised that you don't make any change to your typical caffeine use for 72 hours after the procedure. Since we know caffeine has a major effect on migraines, abruptly quitting caffeine or suddenly increasing your caffeine drinking could have an adverse effect on the results of the treatment.

There are some relative restrictions against any strenuous exercise for the rest of the day after your treatment. If you really have to go exercise, it's probably not going to kill you, but you may not get the best results from your treatment. You may have some temporary numbness in your throat, so be careful when swallowing until the numbness wears off. It is okay for you to drive and do all other normal daily activities after having the RESET treatment.

Can pregnant women have the RESET treatment?

Yes. Both lidocaine and Afrin can be used during pregnancy. You might read on other doctor's websites that the SPG block is not safe during pregnancy. Most likely, this is because these doctors are using x-rays and/or sedation while performing the treatment. You will not need any sedation, any other medications, or be exposed to any radiation for the RESET treatment.

It is common that many non-OB/GYN doctors are very skittish about pregnant women and will generally refuse to do anything to them unless they absolutely have to. Interestingly, migraines will often get better during the second and third trimesters of pregnancy anyway due to hormonal shifts during these times. But even if the headaches don't get better (or get worse) during your pregnancy, it should be safe to have the RESET treatment while pregnant.

Can children have the RESET treatment?

Older kids and teenagers can absolutely have this treatment. Young kids will probably not be able to tolerate it. As a general rule, kids under the age of eight are not going to be able to handle the RESET treatment. Kids over the age of 12 are generally going to be fine having it. Between the ages of 8 and 12, it really depends on the particular child. Some will handle it without any problem, and some will not be able to hold still or cooperate at all. I am always willing to try the treatment for your child, but it is impossible to safely or reliably perform it if the child is not cooperative.

Basically, for your child to have the RESET treatment, he or she needs to be able to hold perfectly still with me looking in their nose with the endoscope and for me to inject the lidocaine into the back of their nose. The lidocaine stings a little when it goes in and it has a yucky chemical flavor. After the medicine goes into the nose, they will need to lie perfectly still while flat on their back for 5-10 minutes afterwards. If you think that your child can handle doing this, then I'm willing to try the RESET treatment for their migraines or other facial pain issues.

How long will the RESET treatment help me?

There's not really any way to know before you try it out. If I were you, I would think first about what your goals are with this treatment. Is your goal to have no headaches at all? Or is it just to have less frequent headaches or less intense headaches? All of these things are potentially possible, but it can vary among different patients. As I stated earlier in this book, about 80-90% of patients will have some amount of benefit for some amount of time after the RESET treatment. Also, 68% of migraine patients will retain some benefit 1 month after the treatment (though that benefit may not be as much as 1 day or 1 week after having the treatment).

Are you already taking medications for migraines or doing any kind of diet or lifestyle changes? All of these things you're already doing have an effect on your migraine threshold and trigger levels. When we start doing the RESET treatment for you, the treatments should also have a positive effect by increasing your migraine threshold. Again, there's no way to know how it's going to work for you unless you try it.

Does the RESET treatment ever stop working?

To my knowledge, the RESET treatment continues to work indefinitely as long as you keep having it done on a regular schedule. People do not become tolerant to the treatment. At the same time, if you stop doing treatments for a while and your symptoms of headache come back, there is no reason you can't start up the RESET treatments again and get back on track.

What if I don't live anywhere near you?

Since you are reading this book, you could certainly be anywhere in the world right now. I would consider contacting some ear, nose and throat doctors (also known as otolaryngologists) in your area and ask them if they perform the sphenopalatine ganglion block to treat migraines. Most likely, they will say they don't perform it, but the SPG block is not a treatment that's terribly complicated for an ear, nose and throat doctor to perform. If you live far away, you can certainly have your doctor contact me and I'd be happy to talk with them and describe my treatment method in more detail. I've filmed a short video on my website for other doctors that describes my experience with the RESET and how I do it. This is at texanent.com/video-for-doctors.

What if I have the procedure and it doesn't help? What if I am in any way unsatisfied with the results?

We know from experience and from the medical literature that somewhere around 80-90% of patients will get some benefit from the RESET treatment. However, that leaves 10-20% who will not have any improvement in their headaches. Because of this fact, I do allow my patients a one week grace period after their first RESET treatment. During this time, you can monitor how you are feeling and if your headaches seem to be getting better or go away completely. If there's no benefit or you're dissatisfied with the benefit, all you need to do is contact my office within 1 week and we will give a refund for the treatment.

It is important to know we will bill you and your insurance for your new patient evaluation, whether or not the RESET treatment works.

How much does the RESET treatment cost?

So far in my practice, everyone has used their health insurance to pay for (or help pay for) the treatment. For a new patient coming to see me for this treatment, there are a couple of different things to keep in mind. First of all, just coming to see me for a new patient evaluation will be billed to your insurance like any other visit to a specialist. The RESET treatment is then billed additionally as a separate procedure charge. It will sometimes be listed on your insurance explanation of benefits as a "surgical procedure" even though it is a simple office treatment.

For billing purposes, my staff will charge for two different billing codes. One is for nasal endoscopy (CPT code 31231) and the other is for sphenopalatine ganglion block (CPT code 64505). You can certainly contact your insurance ahead of time to find out if there's any out of pocket costs for you for each of these codes. The specific details of your insurance plan will determine how much you personally will be responsible for paying. Some patients will pay nothing out of pocket for the RESET treatment and other patients could owe $200 or more depending on their particular insurance plan. My office staff contacts your insurance prior to your visit and will have this payment information available for you at your evaluation with me.

Don't forget that the first time you have the RESET treatment, you have the option of a refund if it doesn't help or if you are dissatisfied with the results after 1 week.

How can I schedule an appointment with you?

My practice is called Texan ENT Specialists. Our main office is in Kyle, Texas, just south of Austin. We also have satellite offices in San Marcos and Lockhart, Texas. You can find out more at our website at texanent.com or call us at 512-550-0321 to make an appointment.

Seth H. Evans, M.D.

Chapter 9:

Let's Wrap This Up

Seth H. Evans, M.D.

9 LET'S WRAP THIS UP

Congrats on making it all the way to the end (well almost). As you've read through this book, you've hopefully learned a lot about migraines and the wide variety of options for their treatment. In the first part of the book, we discussed what most people are doing now and what the "state of the art treatment" is for migraines in the 21st century. You also heard a bit about how migraines happen and what's going on within your brain and your nerves when you're having a migraine.

In the second part of the book, you learned a lot about a "new old" treatment for migraines. You're now an expert on the sphenopalatine ganglion block, its 100 year history, and my spin on this underutilized treatment: the Migraine RESET.

In my opinion, most migraine patients these days are either inadequately treated or wrongly treated. Most of the time, people are self-medicating, but sometimes even their doctors are part of the problem. I believe the goal of migraine treatment should be preventing headaches first and reacting to headaches as a backup plan.

I think that far too often these priorities are reversed and there's no focus at all on prevention of headaches. There are many different ways to prevent migraine headaches by raising your threshold, but a lot of those ways require large amounts of time, willpower and dedication. The Migraine RESET treatment is a relatively painless option that can really have an outsized effect in preventing migraines. If you are a sufferer of frequent migraines, I encourage you to seek out this treatment, whether from me or from another ENT doctor in your area. For more information about myself and my practice, please check out TexanENT.com. There is information for other doctors on my experience and how I perform the RESET treatment at texanent.com/video-for-doctors.

Chapter 10:

Resources

Seth H. Evans, M.D.

10 RESOURCES

Websites: My practice website is texanent.com. If you live in another city and wish to see a local ENT doctor in your area, please ask them to watch the short video at texanent.com/video-for-doctors. This video describes my experience with the RESET treatment and teaches other ENT doctors how to perform it.

Books:

Heal Your Headache by David Buchholz, MD.

This book provides a succinct overview of how most people overuse abortive medications for migraine and wind up in a vicious cycle of rebound headaches. The author provides a one-size-fits-all way to eliminate migraines, which he calls the 1-2-3 program. It is a well-written and informative book, particularly for those who just want to be told what to do to get better. This book was published in 2002, but makes no mention of the sphenopalatine ganglion block.

Migraine Brain by Carolyn Bernstein, MD and Elaine McArdle.

In contrast to the focused 1-2-3 program in Heal Your Headache, this book is much more like an all-you-can-eat buffet with dozens of different treatment options. There is a ton of information in Migraine Brain, but it is well written and it reads quickly. Dr. Bernstein does not name Heal Your Headache specifically, but it is clear that she is laying out some philosophical differences from the recommendations in that book. Migraine Brain was published in 2008, so it is a little more up to date than Heal Your Headache.

Miracles on Park Avenue by Albert Gerber.

This delightful book is a profile of Dr. Milton Reder, an ENT doctor who practiced in New York City from the 1920s through the 1980s. The book details Dr. Reder's successful use of the SPG block for numerous medical conditions, including such conditions as chronic hiccups, erectile dysfunction, and phantom singing noises in the ears. He also treated many types of pain including migraines. The book is out of print, but used copies can be purchased on Amazon.com.

ABOUT THE AUTHOR

Dr. Seth Evans is a born and raised Virginian who realized that he was a Texan at heart after visiting the Austin area a few years ago. After completing his otolaryngology residency in 2010, Dr. Evans spent about half of the next year earning money as a doctor and the other half spending it while he traveled to Australia, New Zealand, Peru, and many parts of Europe. He moved to Central Texas in late 2011 and joined Texan ENT Specialists full time in January 2012.

In his spare time, he enjoys tormenting his friends and family in the north with weather reports of the Texas "winter," attending live music shows, unsuccessfully trying to break 80 on the golf course, stuffing himself with beef brisket, and spending time with his wife, daughter, and 2 Westie dogs.

www.ingramcontent.com/pod-product-compliance
Lightning Source LLC
Chambersburg PA
CBHW030714220526
45463CB00005B/2048